The Best Mediterranean Dessert Recipes for Beginners

A Guide With Delicious Recipes

Dinah D. Johnson

Sommario

Introduction

Thinking about the principle of diet in current times we right away consider radical diet plans such as fasting or ketogenic diet plan, but our publication will certainly offer extra, our publication is based upon fat burning assured with our Mediterranean diet regimen, which is not based on a radical decrease of calories yet at the same time you do not need to give up the swimwear examination.

A false belief of modern-day diets is the impossibility of eating snak or sweets however thanks to this diet plan you will see that it is never so, appreciate delighting in these recipes for you and your family without giving up weight management as well as far better physical strength.

If you are reluctant regarding this great diet you just need to try it and analyze your results in a short time, believe me you will certainly be pleased.

Always remember that the very best method to slim down is to assess your circumstance with the help of a specialist.

Take pleasure in.

Fruity Bread

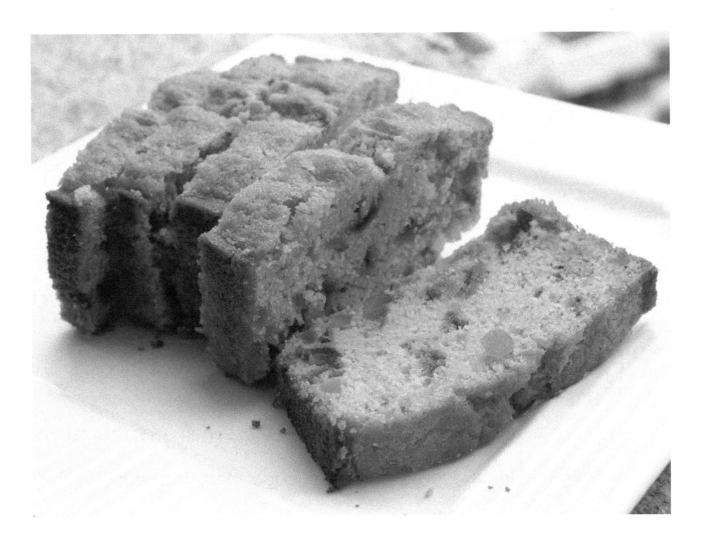

Prep time: 10 minutes I **Cooking time:** 30 minutes I **Servings:**

4

Ingredients:

- 2 cups pears, cored and cubed

- 1 cup coconut sugar

- 2 eggs, whisked

- 2 cups almond flour

- 1 tablespoon baking powder

- 1 tablespoon coconut oil, melted

Directions:

1. In a bowl, mix the pears with the sugar and the other ingredients, whisk, pour into a loaf pan, introduce in the oven and bake at 350 degrees F for 30 minutes.

2. Slice and serve cold.

Nutrition info per serving: calories 380, fat 16.7, fiber 5, carbs 17.5, protein 5.6

Rice Almond Pudding

Prep time: 10 minutes I **Cooking time:** 25 minutes I **Servings:**

4

Ingredients:

- 1 tablespoon avocado oil

- 1 cup brown rice

- 3 cups almond milk

- ½ cup cherries, pitted and halved

- 3 tablespoons coconut sugar

- 1 teaspoon cinnamon powder

- 1 teaspoon vanilla extract

Directions:

1. In a pan, combine the oil with the rice and the other ingredients, stir, bring to a simmer, cook for 25 minutes over medium heat, divide into bowls and serve cold.

Nutrition info per serving: calories 292, fat 12.4, fiber 5.6, carbs 8, protein 7

Watermelon Stew

Prep time: 5 minutes I **Cooking time:** 8 minutes I **Servings:** 4

Ingredients:

- Juice of 1 lime

- 1 teaspoon lime zest, grated

- 1 and ½ cup coconut sugar

- 4 cups watermelon, peeled and cut into large chunks

- 1 and ½ cups water

Directions:

1. In a pan, combine the watermelon with the lime zest, and the other ingredients, toss, bring to a simmer over medium heat, cook for 8 minutes, divide into bowls and serve cold.

Nutrition info per serving: calories 233, fat 0.2, fiber 0.7, carbs

61.5, protein 0.9

Ginger Chia Pudding

Prep time: 1 hour I **Cooking time:** 0 minutes I **Servings:** 4

Ingredients:

- 2 cups almond milk

- ½ cup coconut cream

- 2 tablespoons coconut sugar

- 1 tablespoon ginger, grated

- ¼ cup chia seeds

Directions:

1. In a bowl, combine the milk with the cream and the other ingredients, whisk well, divide into small cups and keep them in the fridge for 1 hour before serving.

Nutrition info per serving: calories 345, fat 17, fiber 4.7, carbs

11.5, protein 6.9

Cashew Cream

Prep time: 2 hours I **Cooking time:** 0 minutes I **Servings:** 4

Ingredients:

- 1 cup cashews, chopped

- 2 tablespoons coconut oil, melted

- 2 tablespoons coconut oil, melted

- 1 cup coconut cream

- 2 tablespoons lemon juice

- 1 tablespoons coconut sugar

Directions:

1. In a blender, combine the cashews with the coconut oil and the other ingredients, pulse well, divide into small cups and keep in the fridge for 2 hours before serving.

Nutrition info per serving: calories 480, fat 43.9, fiber 2.4, carbs 19.7, protein 7

Hemp Cocoa Cookies

Prep time: 30 minutes I **Cooking time:** 0 minutes I **Servings:**

6

Ingredients:

- 1 cup almonds, soaked overnight and drained

- 2 tablespoons cocoa powder

- 1 tablespoon coconut sugar

- ½ cup hemp seeds

- ¼ cup coconut, shredded

- ½ cup water

Directions:

1. In your food processor, combine the almonds with the cocoa powder and the other ingredients, pulse well, press this on a lined baking sheet, keep in the fridge for 30 minutes, slice and serve.

Nutrition info per serving: calories 270, fat 12.6, fiber 3, carbs 7.7, protein 7

Pomegranate Bowls

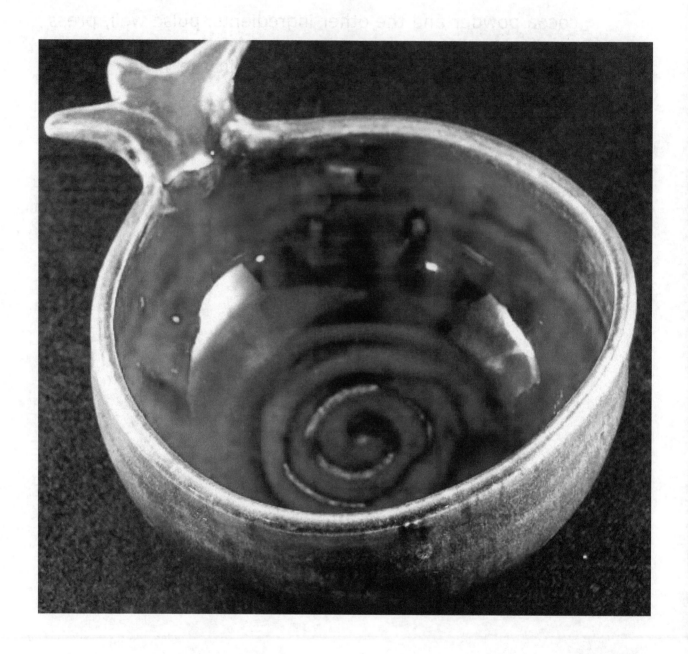

Prep time: 2 hours I **Cooking time:** 0 minutes I **Servings:** 4

Ingredients:

- ½ cup coconut cream

- 1 teaspoon vanilla extract

- 1 cup almonds, chopped

- 1 cup pomegranate seeds

- 1 tablespoon coconut sugar

Directions:

1. In a bowl, combine the almonds with the cream and the other ingredients, toss, divide into small bowls and serve.

Nutrition info per serving: calories 258, fat 19, fiber 3.9, carbs 17.6, protein 6.2

Chia and Blackberries Cream

Prep time: 10 minutes I **Cooking time:** 0 minutes I **Servings:**

6

Ingredients:

- 2 cups coconut cream

- 2/3 cup coconut sugar

- ½ cup blackberries

- 1 cup almond milk

- 3 tablespoons chia seeds, ground

- ½ teaspoon vanilla extract

Directions:

1. In a bowl, combine the cream with the chia seeds and the other ingredients, whisk well, divide into small bowls, leave aside for 10 minutes and serve.

Nutrition info per serving: calories 295, fat 29.2, fiber 3.3, carbs 9.6, protein 3.3

Lime Berries Salad

Prep time: 5 minutes I **Cooking time:** 0 minutes I **Servings:** 4

Ingredients:

- 1 cup blackberries

- 1 cup blueberries

- 1 tablespoon lime juice

- 1 cup strawberries, halved

- 1 tablespoon coconut sugar

- ½ teaspoon ginger powder

- ½ teaspoon vanilla extract

Directions:

1. In a bowl, combine the blackberries with the blueberries and the other ingredients, toss and serve.

Nutrition info per serving: calories 77, fat 0.4, fiber 3.6, carbs 17.4, protein 1.3

Grapefruit Cream

Prep time: 10 minutes I **Cooking time:** 10 minutes I **Servings:**

4

Ingredients:

- 1 cup coconut milk

- 2 tablespoons coconut sugar

- ½ cup coconut cream

- 1 teaspoon vanilla extract

- 4 grapefruits, peeled and roughly chopped

Directions:

1. In a pan, combine the milk with the grapefruits and the other ingredients, whisk, bring to a simmer and cook over medium heat for 10 minutes.

2. Blend using an immersion blender, divide into bowls and serve cold.

Nutrition info per serving: calories 298, fat 21.6, carbs 3.4, fiber 25, protein 3.4

Mango Mix

Prep time: 10 minutes I **Cooking time:** 0 minutes I **Servings:**
4

Ingredients:

- 2 bananas, peeled and sliced

- 2 mangoes, peeled and cubed

- 1 tablespoon walnuts, chopped

- 1 tablespoon lime juice

Directions:

1. In a bowl, combine the bananas with the mangoes and the other ingredients, toss and serve.

Nutrition info per serving: calories 165, fat 2, fiber 4.4, carbs 38.8, protein 2.5

Mango Cream

Prep time: 2 hours I **Cooking time:** 0 minutes I **Servings:** 6

Ingredients:

- 1 watermelon, peeled and cubed

- 1 teaspoon vanilla extract

- ½ teaspoon cinnamon powder

- 2 mangoes, peeled and cubed

Directions:

1. In a blender, combine the watermelon with the mango and the other ingredients, pulse well, divide into bowls and keep in the fridge for 2 hours before serving.

Nutrition info per serving: calories 75, fat 0.5, fiber 1.9, carbs 18.4, protein 1

Cocoa Dates

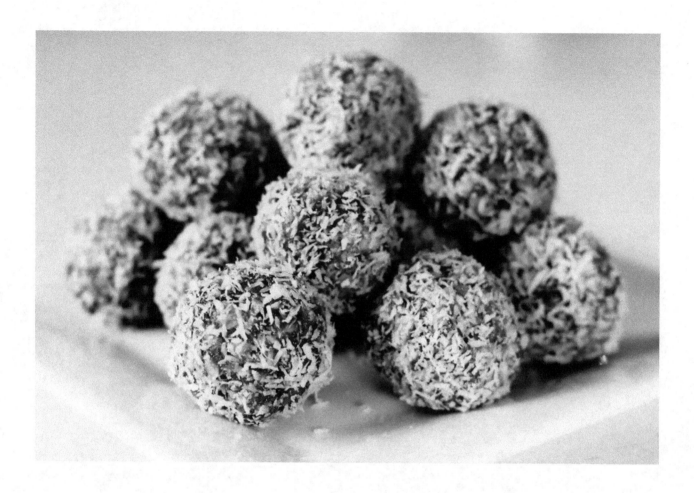

Prep time: 10 minutes I **Cooking time:** 0 minutes I **Servings:**

4

Ingredients:

- 1 cup dates, chopped

- 2 bananas, peeled and sliced

- 1 cup almond milk

- 2 tablespoons cocoa powder

- 1 tablespoon honey

Directions:

1. In a bowl, combine the dates with the bananas and the other ingredients, toss and serve cold.

Nutrition info per serving: calories 338, fat 15, fiber 7.2, carbs 56, protein 3.6

Creamy Apple

Prep time: 10 minutes I **Cooking time:** 0 minutes I **Servings:** 2

Ingredients:

- 2 big green apples, cored and roughly cubed

- 1 tablespoon honey

- 1 cup coconut cream

- 1 teaspoon cinnamon powder

Directions:

1. In a bowl, combine the apples with the cream and the other ingredients, toss and serve.

Nutrition info per serving: calories 100, fat 1, fiber 4, carbs 12, protein 4

Nuts Cream

Prep time: 10 minutes I **Cooking time:** 20 minutes I **Servings:**

6

Ingredients:

- 1 cup pineapple, peeled and cubed

- ½ cup walnuts, chopped

- 1 tablespoon honey

- 1 cup coconut cream

- 1 egg, whisked

- ¼ cup coconut oil, melted

Directions:

1. In a blender, combine the pineapple with the walnuts and the other ingredients, pulse well, divide into 6 ramekins and bake at 370 degrees F for 20 minutes.

2. Serve cold.

Nutrition info per serving: calories 200, fat 3, fiber 4, carbs 12, protein 8

Maple Bars

Prep time: 10 minutes I **Cooking time:** 25 minutes I **Servings:**

6

Ingredients:

- ½ cup coconut cream

- 1 cup apples, peeled, cored and chopped

- ½ cup maple syrup

- 1 teaspoon vanilla extract

- ½ cup almond flour

- 2 eggs, whisked

- 1 teaspoon baking powder

Directions:

1. In a blender, combine the cream with the apples and the other ingredients and pulse well.

2. Pour this into a baking dish lined with parchment paper, bake in the oven at 370 degrees F for 25 minutes, cool down, cut into bars and serve.

Nutrition info per serving: calories 200, fat 3, fiber 4, carbs 12, protein 11

Avocado Salad

Prep time: 10 minutes I **Cooking time:** 0 minutes I **Servings:**

6

Ingredients:

- 3 oranges, peeled and cut into segments

- 1 avocado, peeled, pitted and cubed

- 3 tablespoons raw honey

- ½ teaspoon vanilla extract

- 1 teaspoon orange zest, grated

Directions:

1. In a bowl, combine the oranges with the avocado and the other ingredients, toss and serve.

Nutrition info per serving: calories 211, fat 3, fiber 4, carbs 8,

protein 7

Ginger Apples

Prep time: 10 minutes I **Cooking time:** 30 minutes I **Servings:**

4

Ingredients:

- 2 apples, cored and halved

- 1 tablespoon ginger, grated

- 1 tablespoon turmeric powder

- ¼ cup raw honey

- 1 tablespoon ginger, grated

Directions:

1. Arrange the apples in a baking dish, add the ginger and the other ingredients, and bake at 390 degrees F for 30 minutes.

2. Divide the apples mix between dessert plates and serve.

Nutrition info per serving: calories 90, fat 2, fiber 1, carbs 2, protein 5

Watermelon Cream

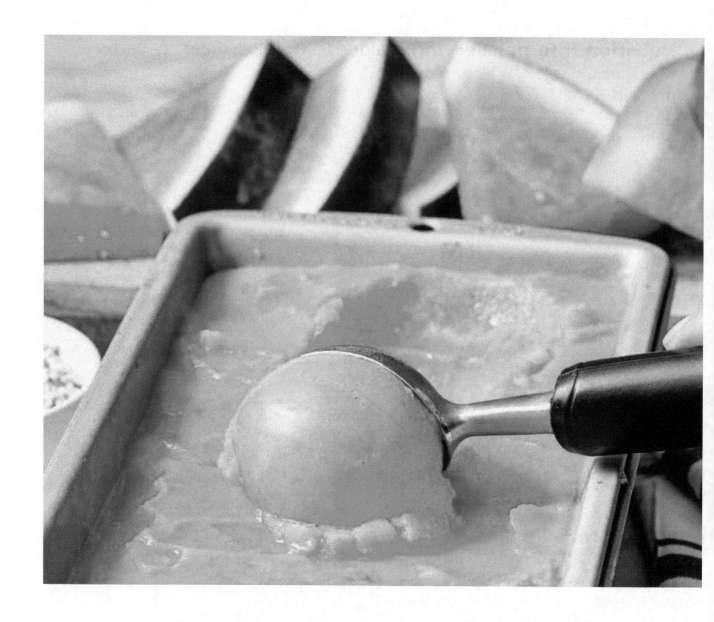

Prep time: 2 hours I **Cooking time:** 0 minutes I **Servings:** 4

Ingredients:

- 2 cups coconut cream

- 1 watermelon, peeled and chopped

- 2 avocados, peeled, pitted and chopped

- 1 tablespoon honey

- 2 teaspoons lemon juice

Directions:

1. In a blender, combine the watermelon with the cream and the other ingredients, pulse well, divide into bowls and keep in the fridge for 2 hours before serving.

Nutrition info per serving: calories 121, fat 2, fiber 2, carbs 6, protein 5

Honey Berry Sorbet

Prep time: 2 hours I **Cooking time:** 0 minutes I **Servings:** 6

Ingredients:

- 1 pound strawberries, halved and frozen

- 1 cup orange juice

- 1 tablespoon orange zest, grated

- 1 tablespoon honey

Directions:

1. In a blender, combine the strawberries with the orange zest and the other ingredients, pulse well, divide into bowls and keep in the freezer for 2 hours before serving.

Nutrition info per serving: calories 121, fat 1, fiber 2, carbs 2, protein 4

Lemony Mix

Prep time: 10 minutes I **Cooking time:** 0 minutes I **Servings:**

4

Ingredients:

- 2 tablespoons almonds, chopped

- 1 tablespoon walnuts, chopped

- 2 cups pineapple, peeled and roughly cubed

- 1 tablespoon lemon juice

- Zest of 1 lemon, grated

- ½ teaspoon vanilla extract

- A pinch of cinnamon powder

Directions:

1. In a bowl, combine the pineapple with the nuts and the other ingredients, toss and serve.

Nutrition info per serving: calories 215, fat 3, fiber 4, carbs 12, protein 8

Cardamom Quinoa Pudding

Prep time: 30 minutes I **Cooking time:** 0 minutes I **Servings:**

4

Ingredients:

- 2 cups almond milk

- 2 tablespoon honey

- 1 cup quinoa, cooked

- A pinch of cardamom powder

- 1 tablespoon lemon zest, grated

Directions:

1. In a bowl, mix the quinoa with the almond milk and the other ingredients, toss, leave aside for 30 minutes, divide into small bowls and serve.

Nutrition info per serving: calories 199, fat 2, fiber 3, carbs 7,

protein 5

Orange Mango Smoothie

Prep time: 10 minutes I **Cooking time:** 0 minutes I **Servings:**

2

Ingredients:

- 2 cups mango, peeled and c hopped

- 1 cup orange juice

- 1 tablespoon ginger, grated

- 1 teaspoon turmeric powder

Directions:

1. In your blender, combine the mango with the juice and the other ingredients, pulse well, divide into 2 glasses and serve cold.

Nutrition info per serving: calories 100, fat 1, fiber 2, carbs 4,

protein 5

Chocolate Cream

Prep time: 2 hours I **Cooking time:** 0 minutes I **Servings:** 4

Ingredients:

- 2 cups coconut milk

- 2 tablespoons ginger, grated

- 2 tablespoons honey

- 1 cup dark chocolate, chopped and melted

- ½ teaspoon cinnamon powder

- 1 teaspoon vanilla extract

Directions:

1. In a blender, combine the coconut milk with the ginger and the other ingredients, pulse well, divide into bowls and keep in the fridge for 2 hours before serving.

Nutrition info per serving: calories 200, fat 3, fiber 5, carbs 12, protein 7

Buttery Avocado Mix

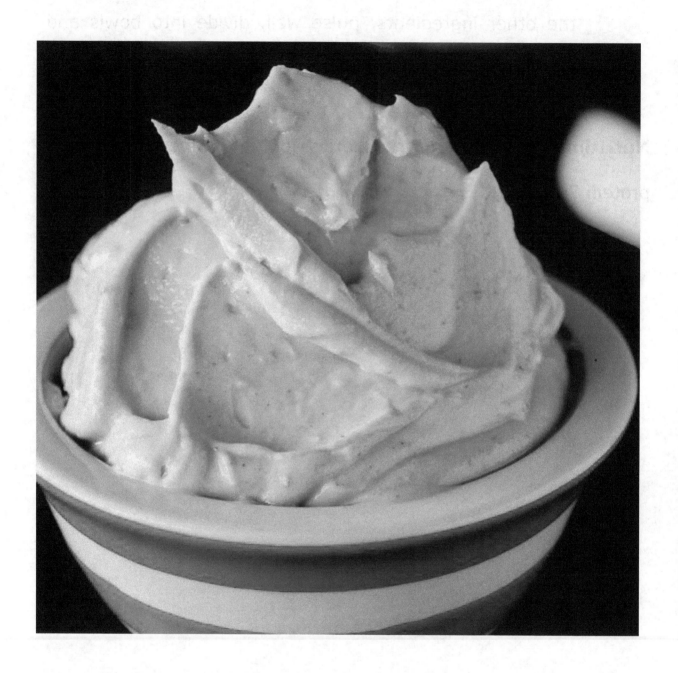

Prep time: 10 minutes I **Cooking time:** 0 minutes I **Servings:**

4

Ingredients:

- 2 avocados, peeled, pitted and cut into wedges

- 1 teaspoon cardamom, ground

- ½ cup coconut butter

- 1 cup coconut cream

- 1 teaspoon vanilla extract

Directions:

1. In your food processor, combine the avocados with the cream and the other ingredients, pulse well, divide into bowls and serve cold.

Nutrition info per serving: calories 211, fat 2, fiber 4, carbs 11, protein 7

Baked Strawberries

Prep time: 10 minutes I **Cooking time:** 20 minutes I **Servings:**

4

Ingredients:

- 1 pound strawberries, halved

- 2 tablespoons almonds, chopped

- 2 tablespoons avocado oil

- 2 tablespoons lime juice

- 1 teaspoon vanilla extract

- 1 teaspoon honey

Directions:

1. Arrange the strawberries on a baking sheet lined with parchment paper, add the almonds and the other ingredients, toss and bake at 390 degrees F for 20 minutes.

2. Divide the strawberries mix into bowls and serve.

Nutrition info per serving: calories 220, fat 2, fiber 3, carbs 8, protein 2

Apple Compote

Prep time: 10 minutes I **Cooking time:** 20 minutes I **Servings:**

4

Ingredients:

- Juice of 1 lime

- 1 pound apples, cored and cut into wedges

- 1 tablespoon honey

- 1 and ½ cups water

Directions:

1. In a pan, combine the apples with the lime juice and the other ingredients, toss, bring to a simmer and cook over medium heat fro 20 minutes.

2. Divide the mix into bowls and serve cold.

Nutrition info per serving: calories 108, fat 1, fiber 2, carbs 4,

protein 7

Vanilla Honey Berries

Prep time: 10 minutes I **Cooking time:** 0 minutes I **Servings:**

4

Ingredients:

- 1 cup blackberries

- 1 cup blueberries

- 2 teaspoons lime zest, grated

- 1 tablespoon raw honey

- ½ teaspoon vanilla extract

- 1 cup almond milk

Directions:

1. In your blender, combine the berries with the lime zest and the other ingredients, pulse well, divide into bowls and serve.

Nutrition info per serving: calories 217, fat 7, fiber 8, carbs 10, protein 8

Maple Coconut Mix

Prep time: 10 minutes I **Cooking time:** 15 minutes I **Servings:**

4

Ingredients:

- 2 cups coconut milk

- 1 cup strawberries

- ¼ teaspoon vanilla extract

- 1/3 cup pure maple syrup

Directions:

1. In a small pot, combine the coconut milk with the berries and the other ingredients, toss, cook over medium heat for 15 minutes, divide into bowls and serve cold.

Nutrition info per serving: calories 176, fat 4, fiber 2, carbs 7,

protein 6

Papaya Bowls

Prep time: 4 minutes I **Cooking time:** 0 minutes I **Servings:** 4

Ingredients:

- 1 cup papaya, roughly cubed

- ½ teaspoon vanilla extract

- 2 tablespoons almonds, chopped

- 1 tablespoon walnuts, chopped

- 2 tablespoons lemon juice

Directions:

1. In a bowl, combine the papaya with the other ingredients, toss, divide into smaller bowls and serve.

Nutrition info per serving: calories 140, fat 1, fiber 2, carbs 3,

protein 5

Orange Squares

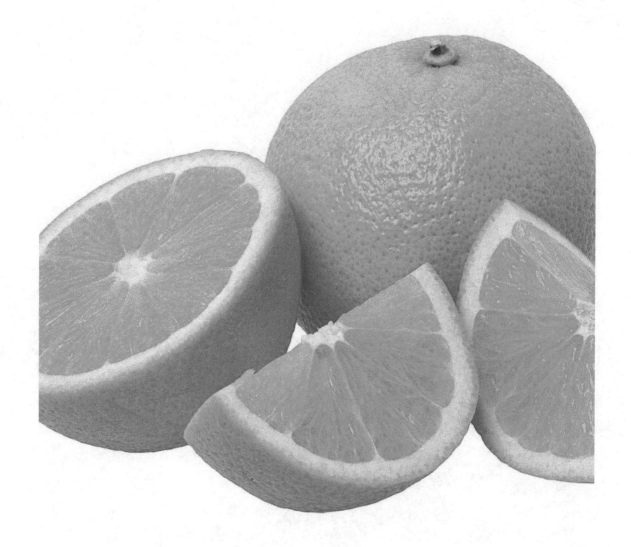

Prep time: 2 hours I **Cooking time:** 0 minutes I **Servings:** 4

Ingredients:

- 1/3 cup natural coconut butter, melted

- 1 and ½ tablespoons avocado oil

- 2 tablespoons orange juice

- ½ teaspoon orange zest, grated

- 1 tablespoons honey

Directions:

1. In a bowl, combine the coconut butter with the oil and the other ingredients, stir well, scoop into a square pan, spread well, cut into squares, keep in the freezer for 2 hours and serve.

Nutrition info per serving: calories 72, fat 4, fiber 2, carbs 8, protein 6

Chia and Honey Mix

Prep time: 10 minutes I **Cooking time:** 0 minutes I **Servings:**

4

Ingredients:

- ¼ cup chia seeds

- 1 cup almond milk

- 2 mangos, peeled and cubed

- 2 teaspoons vanilla extract

- ¼ cup coconut, shredded

- 1 tablespoon honey

Directions:

1. In a bowl, combine the chia seeds with the mango, the milk and the other ingredients, toss, leave aside for 10 minutes, divide into small bowls and serve.

Nutrition info per serving: calories 287, fat 17.2, fiber 5.1, carbs 34.6, protein 3.2

Pomegranate and Berries Mix

Prep time: 2 hours I **Cooking time:** 0 minutes I **Servings:** 4

Ingredients:

- ½ cup coconut cream

- 1 orange, peeled and cut into wedges

- 1 teaspoon vanilla extract

- ½ cup almonds, chopped

- 1 cup pomegranate seeds

- 1 tablespoon orange zest, grated

Directions:

1. In a bowl, combine the orange with the pomegranate seeds and the other ingredients, toss and keep in the

fridge for 2 hours before dividing into smaller bowls and serving.

Nutrition info per serving: calories 68, fat 5.1, fiber 4, carbs 6, protein 1

Almond Bowls

Prep time: 10 minutes

Cooking time: 0 minutes

Servings: 4

Ingredients:

- ½ teaspoon vanilla extract

- 1 cup almonds, chopped

- 1 tablespoon maple syrup

- 1 tablespoon coconut oil, melted

Directions:

1. In a bowl, combine the almonds and the other ingredients, toss, divide into small cups and serve.

Nutrition info per serving: calories 130, fat 5, fiber 5, carbs 12,

protein 4

Apple Mint Cream

Prep time: 10 minutes I **Cooking time:** 0 minutes I **Servings:**

4

Ingredients:

- 1 pounds apples, peeled, cored and cubed

- 2 cups coconut cream

- 1 tablespoon mint, chopped

Directions:

1. In your blender, combine the apples with the cream and mint, pulse well, divide into small cups and serve cold.

Nutrition info per serving: calories 70, fat 9, fiber 3, carbs 4.4, protein 3

Rhubarb Pudding

Prep time: 10 minutes I **Cooking time:** 20 minutes I **Servings:**

6

Ingredients:

- 2 cups rhubarb, sliced

- 2 tablespoons maple syrup

- 3 eggs

- 2 tablespoons coconut oil, melted

- 1 cup almond milk

- ½ teaspoon baking powder

Directions:

1. In a blender, combine the rhubarb with the oil and maple syrup and pulse well.

2. In a bowl, combine the rhubarb puree with the other ingredients, whisk, divide into 6 ramekins and bake at 350 degrees F for 20 minutes.

3. Serve the pudding cold.

Nutrition info per serving: calories 220, fat 12, fiber 3, carbs 7, protein 8

Pears and Dates Cake

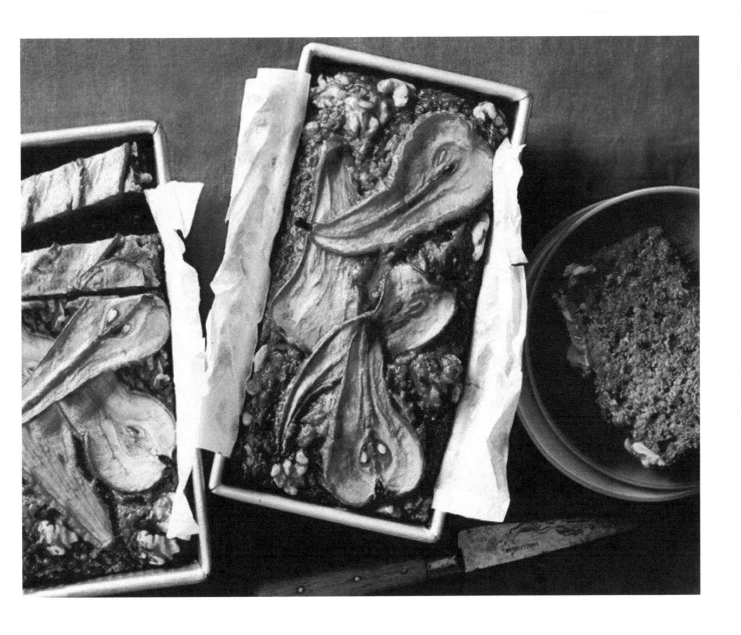

Prep time: 10 minutes I **Cooking time:** 30 minutes I

Servings: 6

Ingredients:

- 2 pears, cored, peeled and chopped

- 2 cups coconut flour

- 1 cup dates, pitted

- 2 eggs, whisked

- 1 teaspoon vanilla extract

- 1 teaspoon baking soda

- ½ cup coconut oil, melted

- ½ teaspoon cinnamon powder

Directions:

1. In a bowl, combine the pears with the flour and the other ingredients, whisk well, pour into a cake pan and bake at 360 degrees F for 30 minutes.

2. Cool down, slice and serve.

Nutrition info per serving: calories 160, fat 7, fiber 4, carbs 8, protein 4

Pears Cream

Prep time: 10 minutes I **Cooking time:** 0 minutes I **Servings:** 4

Ingredients:

- 2 teaspoons lime juice

- 1 pound pears, cored, peeled and chopped

- 1 pound strawberries, chopped

- 1 cup coconut cream

Directions:

1. In a blender, combine the pears with strawberries and the other ingredients, pulse well, divide into bowls and serve.

Nutrition info per serving: calories 100, fat 2, fiber 3, carbs 8, protein 5

Cantaloupe Bowls

Prep time: 10 minutes I **Cooking time:** 0 minutes I **Servings:**

4

Ingredients:

- 1 cantaloupe, peeled and cubed

- 2 tablespoons honey

- 1 cup orange juice

- 1 teaspoon vanilla extract

Directions:

1. In a bowl, combine the cantaloupe and the other ingredients, toss and serve.

Nutrition info per serving: calories 110, fat 2, fiber 3, carbs 6, protein 6

Lime Cherry Cream

Prep time: 10 minutes I **Cooking time:** 15 minutes I **Servings:**

6

Ingredients:

- 1 pound cherries, pitted and chopped

- Juice of 1 lime

- Zest of 1 lime, grated

- 2 tablespoons chicory root powder

- ¼ teaspoon vanilla extract

Directions:

1. In a pot, mix the cherries with the lime juice and the other

   ingredients, toss, simmer over medium heat for 15

minutes, blend using an immersion blender, divide into cups and serve cold.

Nutrition info per serving: calories 120, fat 2, fiber 2, carbs 3, protein 6

Apple and Pear Mix

Prep time: 10 minutes I **Cooking time:** 20 minutes I **Servings:**

6

Ingredients:

- 3 apples, cored and roughly cut into wedges

- 3 pears, cored and cut into wedges

- 4 tablespoons chicory root powder

- 2 teaspoons cinnamon powder

Directions:

1. In a roasting pan, combine the apples with the pears and the other ingredients, toss and cook at 380 degrees F for 20 minutes.

2. Divide the mix between dessert plates and serve.

Nutrition info per serving: calories 110, fat 2, fiber 3, carbs 5, protein 5

Ginger Mango Stew

Prep time: 10 minutes I **Cooking time:** 20 minutes I **Servings:**

4

Ingredients:

- 2 mangoes, peeled and cubed

- 1 tablespoon ginger, grated

- 1 tablespoon cinnamon powder

- 1 teaspoon vanilla extract

- 1 cup water

Directions:

1. In a small pot, combine the mango with the cinnamon and the other ingredients, toss, simmer over medium heat for 20 minutes, divide into bowls and serve.

Nutrition info per serving: calories 140, fat 2, fiber 2, carbs 8,

protein 9

Lime Melon Curd

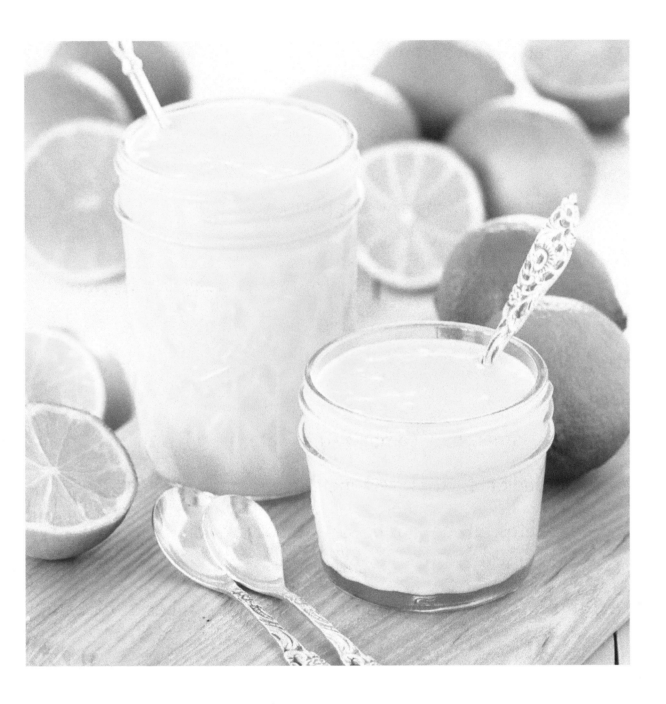

Prep time: 10 minutes I **Cooking time:** 15 minutes I **Servings:**

4

Ingredients:

- 2 tablespoons lime juice

- 2 cups watermelon, peeled and cubed

- 1 tablespoon chicory root powder

- 2 tablespoons flax meal mixed with 4 tablespoons water

Directions:

1. In a small pot, combine the watermelon with the other ingredients, toss, simmer over medium heat for 15 minutes, divide into bowls and serve cold.

Nutrition info per serving: calories 161, fat 4, fiber 2, carbs 8, protein 5

Coconut Papaya Pudding

Prep time: 10 minutes I **Cooking time:** 20 minutes I **Servings:**

4

Ingredients:

- 2 cups coconut milk

- 1 papaya, peeled and chopped

- ½ cup maple syrup

- 3 tablespoons coconut oil, melted

- 3 tablespoons flax meal mixed with 6 tablespoons water

- 1 cup coconut cream

Directions:

1. In your blender, mix the papaya with the coconut milk and the other ingredients, pulse well and divide into 4 ramekins.

2. Place the ramekins in a baking dish, add the water to the dish, introduce in the oven, cook at 350 degrees F for 20 minutes and serve cold.

Nutrition info per serving: calories 171, fat 5, fiber 2, carbs 6, protein 8

Grapes and Walnuts Bowls

Prep time: 10 minutes I **Cooking time:** 15 minutes I **Servings:**

4

Ingredients:

- 2 cups coconut cream

- 1 cup grapes, halved

- 2 cups rolled oats

- 1 teaspoon vanilla extract

- ½ cup walnuts, chopped

Directions:

1. In a small pot, combine the grapes with the cream and the other ingredients, stir, bring to a simmer over medium heat, cook for 15 minutes, divide into bowls and serve cold.

Nutrition info per serving: calories 142, fat 3, fiber 3, carbs 7, protein 4

Papaya Cake

Prep time: 10 minutes I **Cooking time:** 35 minutes I **Servings:**

4

Ingredients:

- 2 cups stevia

- 2 cups coconut flour

- 2 cups papaya, peeled and chopped

- 3 eggs, whisked

- 2 teaspoon baking powder

- 1 teaspoon vanilla extract

- 1 teaspoon nutmeg powder

Directions:

1. In a bowl, combine the stevia with the flour and the other ingredients, whisk well, pour into a cake pan and cover with tin foil.

2. Introduce in the oven, bake at 350 degrees F for 35 minutes, cool it down, slice and serve.

Nutrition info per serving: calories 300, fat 11, fiber 4, carbs 8, protein 4

Quinoa and Blackberry Pudding

Prep time: 10 minutes I **Cooking time:** 35 minutes I **Servings:** 4

Ingredients:

- 3 cups almond milk

- 2 tablespoons chicory root powder

- 1 cup quinoa

- 1 cup blackberries

- 1 tablespoon cinnamon powder

Directions:

1. In a pot, combine the milk with the quinoa and the other ingredients, toss, bring to a simmer over medium-low heat, cook for 35 minutes, divide into bowls and serve cold.

Nutrition info per serving: calories 629, fat 45.7, fiber 9.6, carbs 52.6, protein 10.6

Brown Rice Pudding

Prep time: 10 minutes I **Cooking time:** 30 minutes I **Servings:**

6

Ingredients:

- 1 tablespoon avocado oil

- 1 cup brown rice

- 3 cups almond milk

- 1 cup grapes, chopped

- ½ teaspoon vanilla extract

Directions:

1. In a small pot, combine the rice with the almond milk and

   the other ingredients, stir well, bring to a simmer over

medium heat, cook for 30 minutes, divide into bowls and serve cold.

Nutrition info per serving: calories 172, fat 4, fiber 1, carbs 14, protein 8

Peach Compote

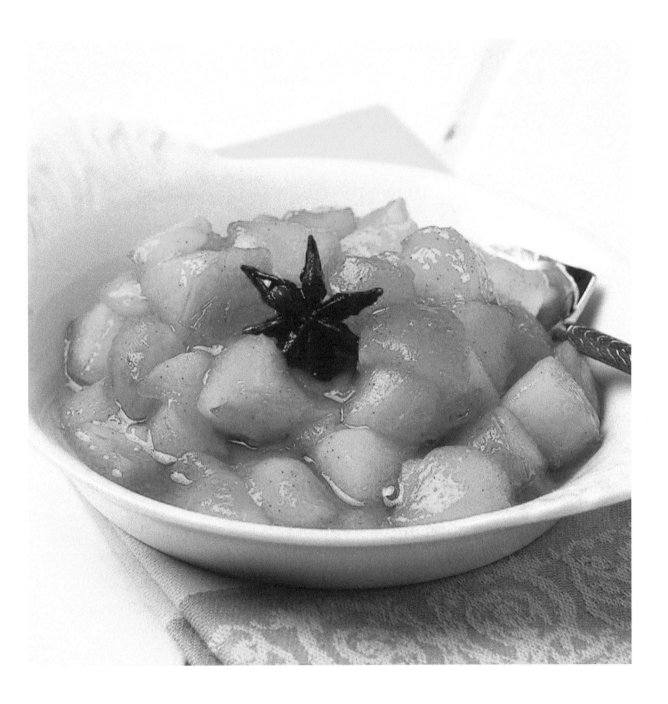

Prep time: 10 minutes I **Cooking time:** 20 minutes I **Servings:**

6

Ingredients:

- 3 peaches, peeled and roughly cubed

- 2 tablespoons chicory root powder

- 1 teaspoon vanilla extract

- 3 cups water

Directions:

1. In a small pot, mix the peaches the other ingredients, stir, bring to a simmer over medium heat, cook for 20 minutes, divide into cups and serve cold.

Nutrition info per serving: calories 122, fat 4, fiber 2, carbs 8, protein 2

Conclusion

Thank you for making it throughout, it would certainly be nice to have responses of your feelings relating to these quick recipes to remain in form without needing to quit the enjoyment of eating your preferred dishes.

Keep in mind that this diet does not just target at slimming yet additionally at physical wellness, try to find the best way to trigger your metabolism, and also remember that this diet plan regimen is an actual anti-aging regimen, the charm of these snak and dessert recipes will certainly allow you to have fun as well as lose weight at the same time and this will allow you to slim down in a tranquil as well as relaxed means without needing to minimize on your own to a situation of anxiety as well as stress.

Have a good time and also enjoy your diet.